Zied CHAARI

Medical and surgical management of Myasthenia Gravis

Zied CHAARI

Medical and surgical management of Myasthenia Gravis

ScienciaScripts

Imprint

Any brand names and product names mentioned in this book are subject to trademark, brand or patent protection and are trademarks or registered trademarks of their respective holders. The use of brand names, product names, common names, trade names, product descriptions etc. even without a particular marking in this work is in no way to be construed to mean that such names may be regarded as unrestricted in respect of trademark and brand protection legislation and could thus be used by anyone.

Cover image: www.ingimage.com

This book is a translation from the original published under ISBN 978-620-6-70872-8.

Publisher:
Sciencia Scripts
is a trademark of
Dodo Books Indian Ocean Ltd. and OmniScriptum S.R.L publishing group

120 High Road, East Finchley, London, N2 9ED, United Kingdom
Str. Armeneasca 28/1, office 1, Chisinau MD-2012, Republic of Moldova, Europe
Printed at: see last page
ISBN: 978-620-7-40400-1

INTRODUCTION

Myasthenia gravis (MG) is an autoimmune disease affecting the neuromuscular junction, responsible for the production of autoantibodies against acetylcholine receptors in striated skeletal muscle. This damage is responsible for the appearance of fluctuating muscle fatigue which, when generalised, could be life-threatening.Autoimmune myasthenia must be distinguished from other myasthenic syndromes, including congenital myasthenia, myasthenia of toxic or drug origin, and Lambert Eaton's myasthenic syndrome of paraneoplastic origin, secondary to the presence of antibodies to pre-synaptic voltage-dependent calcium channels.The origin of the immune dysfunction is still unknown, but the presence of immune dysregulation associated with thymic abnormalities plays an important role in the pathogenesis of this disease [1]. The association of myasthenia seen in thymic pathology was first described in 1901 by Laquer on an autopsy of a patient who had died following myasthenia and in whom he discovered a thymic tumour [2].

Medical treatment (mainly including drugs to increase neuromuscular transmission, immunosuppressants, immunoglobulins, monoclonal antibodies or plasma exchange) is often combined with surgical management to perform a simple or enlarged thymectomy. Described for the first time in 1939 by Blalock et al [3], thymectomy for MG has become the surgical standard for the treatment of this condition, giving patients twice the chance of complete withdrawal of medical treatment.At present, it is generally accepted that surgical thymectomy should be proposed for all patients with MG (thus enabling

 The only exception is patients with positive anti-MuSK antibodies, in whom surgery is still ineffective [4-6].

Myasthenia Gravis is an autoimmune disease linked to a blockage of receptors located in the motor plate of skeletal muscles by anti-acetylcholine receptor antibodies. Clinically, this blockage manifests itself as excessive fatigability of the striated muscle, which improves with rest or after the use of anti-cholinesterase drugs.

Myasthenia, like any other autoimmune disease, involves several pathogenic factors responsible for the ultimate production of autoantibodies directed against motor plate molecules, leading to disruption of the normal functioning of neuromuscular transmission (Figure 1).

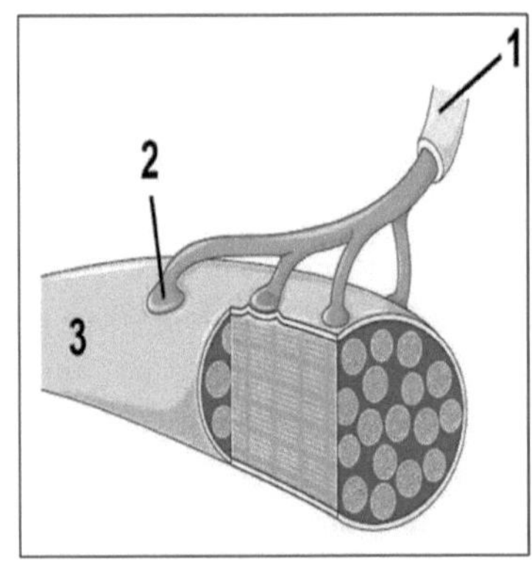

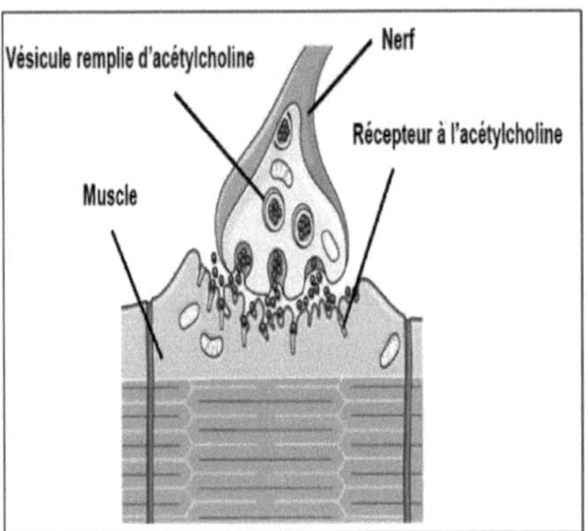

Figure 1: Skeletal muscle motor plate

1. EPIDEMIOLOGY

Myasthenia gravis is a disease that occurs in both sexes and at all ages. The incidence of this disease varies according to studies and series. It ranges from 1.7 to 21.3/1,000,000 of the population, with a prevalence that varies as widely between 43 and 64 / 1,000,000 population [7, 8]. In France, this condition is more or less rare, with an estimated overall incidence of between 2 and 5 cases/1,000,000 population [9]. Some studies have reported a predominance of women, especially before the age of 50 (up to 60 or 70%), whereas this difference diminishes after the age of 50. In their 10-year series (1990-2000), Aragones et al [10] reported an overall incidence of myasthenia at 21.27 cases/1,000,000 population. The incidence described increased from 5.03/1,000,000 inhabitants in young people under the age of 15, to 14.68/1,000,000 inhabitants in patients aged between 15 and 64, to 63.38/1,000,000 inhabitants in patients aged over 64. This study also reported a clear male predominance after the age of 60, in patients presenting with myasthenia distinct from that associated with thymomas. Clinically, the first signs are purely ocular in almost 50% of cases (ptosis and/or diplopia), with other muscle areas being affected after one year in more than 80% of patients (respiratory, limb, pharyngeal and laryngeal muscles affected), subsequently forming the procession of generalised myasthenia gravis. Myasthenia can remain localised to the eye in less than 20% of cases, forming ocular myasthenia. In this case, generalisation is still rare and occurs late.

2. PATHOPHYSIOLOGY

The pathophysiology of myasthenia has been clarified several times in recent years, and essentially involves two major factors: the thymus and pathogenic antibodies.

a- Role of the thymus: This role has been incriminated in the pathology of myasthenia following several experimental evidences:

✓ The efficacy of surgical thymectomy in the treatment and improvement of clinical symptomatology in myasthenics with the frequency of histological types of surgical excisions.

✓ Production of specific anti-human acetylcholine receptor antibodies following injection of human myasthenic thymic tissue into mice.

✓ The thymus shows hyperplasia (development of germinal centres housing B lymphocytes with a border of T lymphocytes) in almost 50% of myasthenic women who secrete anti-acetylcholine receptor antibodies. This entity is often associated with HLAB8 DR3.

✓ Expression of the acetylcholine receptor in thymic B and T lymphocytes, with the possibility of local intra-thymic synthesis of anti-receptor antibodies.

✓ Certain viral infections that can affect the functioning of the thymus, in particular Epstein Bar Virus (EBV).

✓ The absence of thymic involution beyond the age of 40, with the development in 20% of patients of a thymic tumour or thymoma, essentially characterised by disorganisation of the cellular architecture, with abnormal overexpression on tumour cells of acetylcholine receptor epitopes and striated muscle antigens, and a reduction in the number of thymic regulatory cells. These changes will subsequently lead to a defect in thymocyte selection, favouring the formation of cells sensitised to acetylcholine receptors and subsequently predisposing to myasthenia.

b- Role of pathogenic antibodies :

✓ Anti-acetylcholine receptor antibodies: these antibodies are directed against acetylcholine receptors and measured by immunoprecipitation. These antibodies lead to a reduction in the number of acetylcholine receptors and a subsequent reduction in the safety margin at the neuromuscular junction. They are generally positive in 75% of generalised myasthenias and 50% of ocular myasthenias. Three different mechanisms of action of these antibodies have been described:

•Destruction of the post-synaptic membrane by complement

•Presence of a block at the acetylcholine binding site itself

•Antigenic modulation responsible for accelerated degradation of membrane acetylcholine receptors.

The greater the number of receptors affected, the worse the prognosis for myasthenia. The prognosis is therefore not correlated with the level of anti-acetylcholine receptor antibodies, nor with the location of the epitopes recognised by the antibodies on the receptor constituents. It is correlated with the presence of a thymoma, except in elderly subjects.

✓ Anti-MUSK antibodies: MuSK is a post-synaptic tyrosine phosphokinase molecule involved in the transcription of acetylcholine receptors and its membrane anchoring. These antibodies are present in 4% of patients with generalised myasthenia without the presence of anti-receptor antibodies.

✓ Other antibodies: some forms of generalised myasthenia do not present anti-receptor or anti-MUSK antibodies. These are known as "negative" myasthenias and are secondary to other antibodies recently detected by immunostaining on embryonic kidney cells, namely

•Anti-acetylcholine receptor antibodies of low affinity

•Anti-RLP4 antibodies: an Arginine receptorwhi ch activates the MuSK

c- Genetic predisposition in myasthenia (Figures 2, 3): Familial forms of myasthenia remain rare. However, associations between early forms of myasthenia with thymic hyperplasia and HLA-DR3 (MHC class II) and HLA-B8 (MHC class I) alleles have been reported in several studies [9, 11].

For early forms of myasthenia, an association with the HLA-DR3 allele has been demonstrated. This allele appears to have a protective role in late forms of the disease. Furthermore, a particular TNF (Tumor Necrosis Factor) allele associated with high production of TNFα, as well as a gene called TNIP1, have been incriminated in women with early myasthenia [12, 13].

For late forms of myasthenia, a role inverse to that of the HLA-DR3 allele has been demonstrated for the HLA-DR7 allele, which seems to be protective in early myasthenia and incriminated in late myasthenia. For patients with myasthenia with anti-MusK antibodies, an association has been established between the disease and HLA-DR14-DQ5 molecules [9].

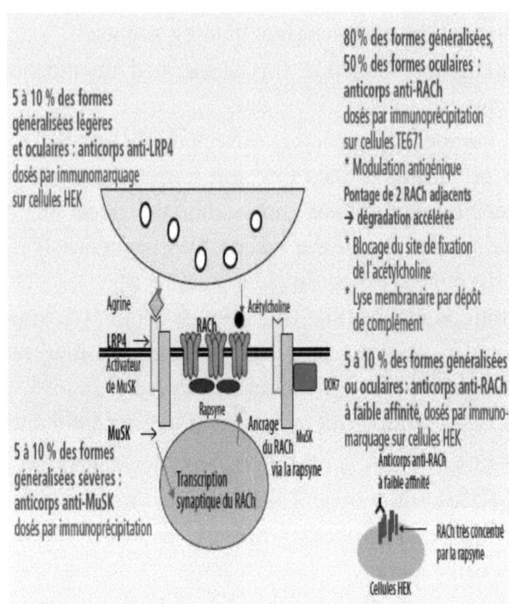

Figure 2: Antibodies specific to autoimmune myasthenia [14].

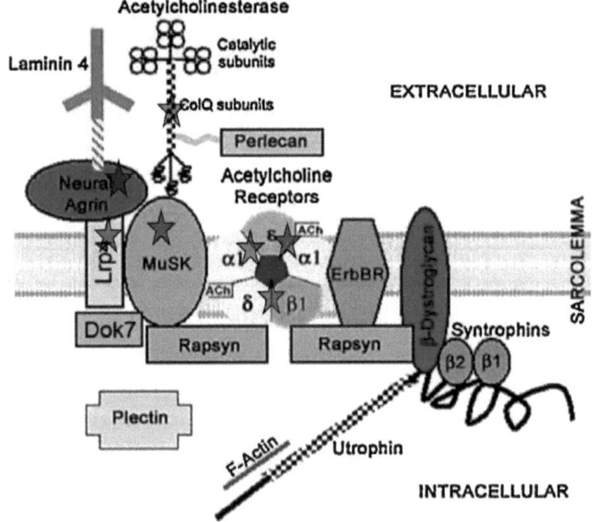

Figure 3: Schematic representation of neuromuscular junction molecules with targets of autoantibody attack (star) [9].

3. CLINICAL PRESENTATION

The onset of clinical manifestations of myasthenia can be either sudden or insidious. It varies from one patient to another, from one time of year to another, and according to the rhythm of the day, with symptoms essentially worsening with muscular effort.

Clinical signs generally combine, to varying degrees, disorders of the :

✓ eye muscles (responsible for diplopia and/or ptosis)

✓ facial muscles

✓ of the muscles of swallowing: causing false routes with sometimes dysphagia develops

✓ of the laryngeal muscles: with the onset of phonatory problems dysphonia, or a nasal airway.

✓ chewing muscles: appearance of a hanging jaw

✓ neck muscles: leading to an inability to raise the head (head drooping)
✓ limb muscles: this is usually asymmetric, and may be proximal (affecting the shoulder muscles, causing difficulty in lifting the upper limbs) or distal (affecting the fingers and hands, causing difficulty in writing and manual work). When the muscles of the lower limbs are affected, the legs become very tired, making it difficult to stand up or sit down, which can sometimes be disabling.
✓ respiratory muscles: this is a serious factor in the progression of the disease, and could be life-threatening for patients.

The clinical evaluation of myasthenia involves several scores as well as additional biological and/or functional tests, including :
- **The MGFA (Myasthenia Gravis Foundation of America) score**: The Myasthenia Gravis Foundation of America (MGFA) clinical classification is intended to identify subgroups of MG with different clinical signs or severity:
o Class I: eye muscle deficit. May have weakness of

occlusion of the eyes. The strength of all other muscles is normal

o Class II: discrete deficit of muscles other than the ocular muscles. May have ocular muscle deficits of any severity:
▪ Class IIa: predominantly affecting limb or axial muscles ;
▪ Class IIb: predominantly affecting the oropharyngeal or respiratory muscles
o Class III: moderate deficit of muscles other than the ocular muscles. May

have an eye muscle deficit of any severity:
- Class IIIa: predominantly affecting limb or axial muscles
- Class IIIb: predominantly affecting the oropharyngeal or respiratory muscles
o Class IV: severe deficit of muscles other than the ocular muscles. May have an eye muscle deficit of any severity:
- Class IVa: predominantly affecting limb or axial muscles ;
- Class IVb: predominantly affecting the oropharyngeal or respiratory muscles
o Class V: need for intubation.

- **The MGFA score after surgery or post-operatively**: is generally used to assess the patient's progress and clinical condition after resection of the thymus and mediastinal fat.

o Score 1: Stable complete remission: no signs or symptoms of myasthenia for at least one year, no treatment. Examination: no weakness, isolated eyelid weakness accepted.

o Score 2: Pharmacological remission: same as 1 except continued treatment

o Score 3: Minimal manifestation: The patient has no symptoms of functional limitation due to myasthenia, but has some weakness on examination of a few muscles.

o Score 4: Improved: A substantial reduction in the symptoms noted before treatment, or a substantial and lasting reduction in the treatment of myasthenia gravis.

o Score 5: Unchanged: No substantial change in the clinical manifestations present before treatment or reduction in the treatment of myasthenia gravis.

o Score 6: Worsening: Substantial increase in clinical manifestations noted before treatment or increase in myasthenia treatments.

o Score 7: Relapse: The patient has met the criteria for stable complete remission, pharmacological remission or minimal manifestations, but subsequently develops more significant clinical signs than those permitted by these criteria.

- **Osserman muscular strength score**: The Osserman score includes a score for muscular strength of the limbs as well as the muscles of the head, oculomotor, chewing, swallowing and phonation. A score is awarded according to the degree of muscular damage and weakness of movement caused. The Osserman score is shown in the figure below:

• Tenue des bras tendus (épreuve de Barré) 10 sec=1pt	150 s = 15 pts
• Tenue des jambes levées (épreuve de Mingazzini) 5 sec=1pt	75 s = 15 pts
• Possibilité de soulever la tête du lit	
Avec contre pression	10 pts
Seulement sans contre pression	5 pts
Non	0 pt
• Possibilité de se relever du décubitus sans aide des bras	
Oui	10 pts
Non	0 pt
• Paralysie oculomotrice	
Aucune	10 pts
Ptosis isolé	5 pts
Ophtalmoplégie	0 pt
• Occlusion palpébrale	
Normale	10 pts
Diminuée	7 pts
Incomplète avec recouvrement cornéen	5 pts
Incomplète sans recouvrement cornéen	0 pt
• Mastication	
Normale	10 pts
Faible	5 pts
Nulle	0 pt
• Déglutition	
Normale	10 pts
Difficile	5 pts
Fausse route	0 pt
• Phonation	
Normale	10 pts
Nasonnée	5 pts
Impossible	0 pt
	Total = 100 pts

Figure 4: Schematic representation of the molecules in the

- **Autoantibody tests**: anti-acetylcholine, anti-muscle specific tyrosine kinase (muSK), anti-nuclear, anti-thyroid, SSA, SSB, rheumatoid factors, anti-phospholipids, ANCA, HLAB27.

Myasthenia can be classified into several subclasses according to the age of onset of symptoms, the clinical presentation, whether or not it is associated with a thymic tumour, and the presence or absence of autoantibodies, all of which are directed against neuromuscular junction proteins in the motor plate.

3.1. Clinical form of myasthenia with antibody to acetylcholine

In this form, three types of clinical presentation can be distinguished according to age of onset :

3.1.1. Neonatal form

Described in myasthenic mothers with the possibility of passage of anti-acetylcholine receptor autoantibodies across the placental membrane causing neonatal myasthenia.

3.1.2. Early onset before the age of 50

This clinical form is more common in women and is associated with thymic hyperplasia. The role of female sex hormones has been incriminated in the pathophysiology of this clinical form, which is frequently associated with other autoimmune pathologies: thyroiditis, which should be systematically investigated.

3.1.3. The late form over 50

This form is generally severe and generalised, associated with bulbar signs and frequent attacks of myasthenia. It is often associated with a thymic tumour (thymoma). Autoantibody testing may reveal autoantibodies to striated muscle proteins such as titin and Ryanodin.

3.2. Form of myasthenia with anti-MUSK antibodies

This form is characterised by the presence of generalised myasthenia with the absence of anti-acetylcholine receptor antibodies in 40% of cases. Hence the importance of testing for anti-MUSK antibodies in myasthenia with negative anti-receptor antibodies. It generally affects young women, with respiratory, bulbar and facial muscle involvement. Ocular signs are rarely observed, and there is no associated thymic pathology (neither thymic hypertrophy nor thymic tumour).

3.3. Clinical form with anti RLP4 antibodies

This clinical form has been identified in 20% of patients with generalised myasthenia gravis with negative anti-acetylcholine receptor and anti-MuSK autoantibodies. This form was first described in 2011 by Higuchi et al [15] but the particularities of the clinical presentation have not been specified, nor has its association with a possible thymic pathology.

3.4. Clinical form without antibodies or seronegative form

These are clinical forms in which the myasthenia can be either generalised or purely ocular, with the absence of all antibodies (anti-acetylcholine receptor, anti-MUSK and anti-RLP4) on further examination. This seronegative form is often secondary to the non-detection of anti-acetylcholine receptor antibodies anchored to the cell surface, but not detected by conventional tests. The clinical forms of MG and their characteristics are summarised in Table I :

Table I: Clinical forms of myasthenia gravis and their clinical and paraclinical characteristics

Clinical form	Early form (<50 years old)	Late form (> 50 years old)	Myasthenia gravis MuSK (+)	Myasthenia RLP4 (+)	Myasthenia Negative
Gender	Women	Female = Men	Women	Unknown	Unknown
Thymus	Hyperplasia	Thymoma	Normal	Unknown	Hyperplasia
Myasthenia	No (Eye signs)	Severe and widespread	Severe and generalised (bulbar, face), respiratory)	widespread	Pure or generalised ocular
Autoimmune diseases	frequently associated	No	No	Unknown	No
Anti-acetylcholine receptor antibodies	+++	+++	-	-	-
Anti-MUSK antibodies	-	-	+	-	-
Anti-RLP4 antibodies	-	-	-	+	
Genetic factors	HLA-DR3	HLA-B7 DR2 TNF allele (TNFα++) TNIP1 gene	HLA-DR14 HLA-DQ5 HLA-DR16		

4. DIFFERENTIAL DIAGNOSIS

They include all pathologies that may mimic myasthenia as well as other myasthenic syndromes [16, 17].

4.1. Ptosis:

We need to eliminate
- Blepharospasm: symmetrical contracture of the orbicularis muscles of both eyelids with facial hemi-spasm, palpebral contracture and syncinesia.

- Claude Bernard Horner syndrome: a combination of ptosis, miosis and enophthalmos secondary to damage to the first sympathetic root.

- Senile ptosis: drooping of the upper eyelid in connection with age. It is moderate and bilateral.

- Involvement of the third cranial nerve: associated with ptosis and homolateral involvement of the superior rectus, medial rectus and lesser oblique.
- Cavernous sinus meningioma: ptosis, homolateral involvement of the oculomotor and V nerves.

4.2. Diplopia :

Multiple sclerosis is most likely in young adults with optic neuritis, vestibular, cerebellar and pyramidal syndromes with hyper-signals on MRI.

4.3. Oculomotor muscle involvement :

✓ Graves' disease: associated with an inflammatory red eye andexophthalmos. However, Graves' disease may be associated with myasthenia gravis [18].
✓ Guillain-Barré polyradiculoneuritis: associated with oculomotor disorders, deficits of the face and limbs, and swallowing disorders. This syndrome is generally associated with sensory disorders, areflexia and albuminocyte dissociation on lumbar puncture.

✓ Miller Fisher syndrome: ophthalmoplegia, ataxia with presence of anti-ganglioside antibodies.

✓ Ocular myopathy: significant ophthalmoplegia not associated with diplopia.

4.4. Bulbar disorders :

✓ Cerebrovascular accident: acute onset

✓ Amyotrophic lateral sclerosis: fasciculations, muscular atrophy, progressive onset, dysarthria and pyramidal damage.

4.5. Other myasthenic syndromes :

✓ Lambert Eaton syndrome: pre-synaptic disease secondary to presence of anti-calcium channel antibodies

✓ Congenital myasthenic syndrome: 10-20% of newborns born to myasthenic mothers present with neonatal myasthenia. This is a transient myasthenic syndrome due to the trans-placental passage of anti-acetylcholine receptor antibodies, more rarely anti-MuSK antibodies.

✓ Botulism: a syndrome following the ingestion of canned food or injected heroin.

✓ Iatrogenic myasthenic syndrome [19]: secondary to chloroquine, D-Penicillamine, hydroxychloroquine, interferons and anti- TNF Alpha.

5. DISEASE ASSESSMENT AND ADDITIONAL TESTS

When faced with a syndrome of muscular weakness, given the multitude of differential diagnoses with myasthenia, a physical examination and detailed questioning are essential in order to make a positive diagnosis. Additional tests are then carried out to confirm and support the suspected diagnosis. They include :

5.1. Testing for anti-acetylcholine receptor antibodies:

It is a mandatory test for all patients with suspected myasthenia. This test has a sensitivity of between 70 and 95% for myasthenia gravis and between 50 and 75% for ocular myasthenia [20]. However, the value of these antibodies does not correlate with the severity of the disease. An additional anti-MuSK antibody test is indicated if the anti-acetylcholine receptor antibody test is negative [21]. Seronegative patients may seroconvert, which is estimated at 15% per year. Concomitant immunotherapy treatment may be the cause of seronegativity to autoantibodies.

5.2. Neurophysiological tests :

Repeated nerve stimulation (RNS) and EMG are the neurological tests most commonly used to diagnose myasthenia. The results of these tests may be erroneous under anti-cholinesterase treatment, which should be stopped a week before the tests.

With regard to SNR: stimulation at 3-10 hertz typically produces a progressive decrease in the amplitude of the muscle action potential. This test is generally positive in 80% of patients with generalised myasthenia gravis and in 50% of patients with ocular myasthenia. The specificity of this test varies according to the type of nerve tested [22].

For the EMG :

Electro-physiological examination reveals neuromuscular block. The motor nerve is stimulated at a frequency of 3 Hertz and the amplitude of the muscular response or motor potential is recorded according to the excitation threshold. In myasthenia, the disturbance in neuromuscular transmission is responsible for a decrease in the amplitude of the motor potential or a decrease in the amplitude of the neuromuscular potential.decrement > 10%. The search for decrement should be carried out, if possible in the absence of anti-cholinesterase treatment, on several nerve-muscle pairs such as the facial, spinal, ulnar and radial nerves, giving priority to symptomatic areas. Diagnostic sensitivity does not exceed 75% and, when the block is lacking, a single-fibre examination can be carried out, which is more complex to perform and only carried out in a few centres, and which can show a prolongation of the response of two muscle fibres of the same motor unit during voluntary effort.This test is the most sensitive in the course of myasthenia and should be performed if neuromuscular junction disease is suspected or if the SNR test is negative. EMG has an estimated sensitivity of 99% in severe generalised myasthenia and 80% in ocular myasthenia [23]. Like the SNR test, the specificity of EMG is variable and may be abnormal in cases of mitochondrial cytopathies, radiculopathies or other nerve diseases.

5.3. Anti-cholinesterase test :

It is a test designed to assess the reversibility of muscle fatigue under short-acting ainti-cholinesterase treatment. This test has a sensitivity of 88% for generalised MG, 92% for ocular myasthenia, and a specificity of 97% for both clinical forms [24].This test should be avoided, especially in elderly subjects, because of the risk of extreme bradycardia and cardiac arrest, hence the need for prophylactic administration of atropine before it is carried out.

- **Prostigmine test**

o Contraindications:

▪Respiratory failure/distress

▪Asthma

▪Mechanical obstruction of the digestive and urinary tracts

▪Known allergy

o Precautions for use

▪Doing an ECG

▪Prepare Prostigmine: 1 mg or 2 x 0.5 mg ampoules

▪Prepare 0.5 mg of atropine

▪CI to atropine :

- Glaucoma

- Prostate adenoma

- Rhythm disorders

- Chronic bronchitis

▪ Objectively assess the motor deficit: myasthenic score, oculomotricity, etc.
o Test procedure :

▪ Slow IV injection of 0.25 mg atropine

▪ Inject 1/4 of the dose (Prostigmine or placebo) IV

▪ Check tolerance (absence of muscarinic signs)

▪ Inject the rest of the dose in 30 seconds

▪ Repeat the test with the other product (placebo or Prostigmine)

o The effect is slow (10 to 15 minutes) and lasts 1 to 2 hours (may last longer in the case of concomitant treatment with corticosteroids).
o Tolerance :

▪ Slow IV injection of 0.25 mg atropine in the event of poor performance.

tolerance :

- Sweats

- Excessive salivation, tears

- Bradycardia++, hypotension.

- Repeat the injection if necessary.

- **Glucagon test:** The ice cube test consists of looking for a reduction in ptosis after applying an ice cube to the eyelid for 1 minute. The test is considered positive if it results in an increase of at least 2 mm in the palpebral slit; this improvement generally lasts less than 1 minute. It is important to observe the patient for 1 to 2 minutes after the test, as correction of the ptosis may be slightly delayed. The positivity of this test is a major argument for the diagnosis of myasthenia, as its sensitivity is close to 95% for ocular myasthenias and its specificity is evaluated at 97%. Pre-therapeutic assessments prior to the proposal for curative surgery: possible immunoglobulins, plasmapheresis sessions, optimal doses of anti-cholinesterase to balance the disease.

▪ The need for plasma exchange (PE) sessions or not, as well as their pre-op numbers

▪ The need to administer immunoglobulins pre-operatively

▪ Preoperative treatment with Mestinon, as well as the dose necessary to balance the symptoms.

5.4. Ice cube test :

This test consists of placing an ice cube over the eyelids for two minutes in order to differentiate between ptosis secondary to myasthenia gravis with neuromuscular transmission disorder (improvement of ptosis in this case) and that secondary to other causes. This test has a sensitivity of 89% and a specificity of 100% [25].

5.5. Testing for anti-Muscle Specific Kinase (MuSK) antibodies:

Testing for anti-MUSK antibodies has been proposed for patients with seronegative MG with negative anti-acetylcholine receptor antibodies. In their series of 78 patients, Evoli et al. reported that the level of anti-MUSK antibodies correlated with the clinical presentation of seronegative myasthenia gravis (anti-acetylcholine receptor antibodies negative). According to this study, patients responded well to pharmacological treatment, although some patients had disease refractory to the usual treatments, with myasthenia gravis unresponsive to the various anti-cholinesterase agents and immunosuppressants [26].

5.6. Imaging and myasthenia :

5.6.1. Chest X-ray :

Given the retro-sternal mediastinal location of the thymic pathology that may be associated with myasthenia, the thoracic X-ray plays a minor role in radiological diagnosis, due to its poor accuracy. It would be useful in myasthenia associated with a thymic tumour (a mediastinal opacity could be demonstrated in this case) [27]. Given the frequent association of MG with the possible presence of underlying thymic hyperplasia or thymic tumour, every patient should benefit from a thoracic CT scan or magnetic resonance imaging (MRI).

5.6.2. Chest computed tomography (CT) :

This is the examination of choice in mediastinal pathology. It will look for a focal density abnormality in the thymic cavity (Figure 5). However, differentiation between a small thymoma and lymphoid hyperplasia of the thymus is difficult. is not always possible [27]. Nevertheless, regular monitoring by chest CT scan is recommended, even in cases of stabilised myasthenia, in order to rule out the presence of a thymoma, which could occur late in the course of the disease (Figure 6).

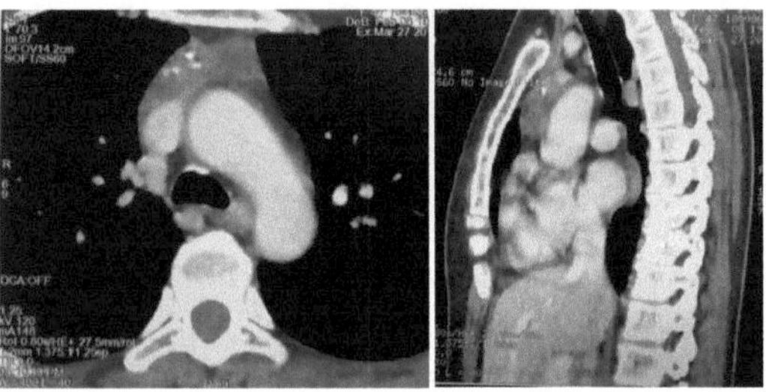

Figure 5: Transverse and coronal sections in the mediastinal window showing a mass in the thymic cavity associated with clinical MG (Thymoma).

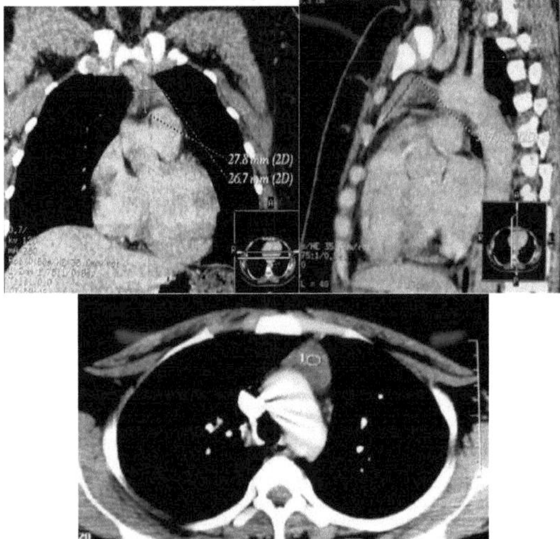

Figure 6: Transverse, frontal and coronal CT sections in the mediastinal window showing a mass in the thymic cavity.

5.6.3. Thoracic MRI :

MRI is not generally used to diagnose myasthenia. However, it is useful in differentiating between thymoma and thymic hyperplasia. Differentiation is easier on MRI than on thoracic CT (94% versus 83% for CT), especially when chemical shift sequences are used [28]. In addition, diffusion-weighted MRI can differentiate between lipid-poor thymus, hyperplastic thymus and thymoma. It is also useful for differentiating between early and advanced thymomas. [27].

5.6.4. Positron emission tomography (PET) :

This examination is not routinely used in myasthenia, but it is useful in differentiating between thymoma and thymic carcinoma. Mineo et al. reported in their series that in myasthenia, fixation was higher (in the thymus and perithymic tissues) than in non-myasthenic or non-neoplastic patients. The Standardized Uptake Value (SUV) was statistically correlated with the presence of thymic germinal centres in the thymus, and with the presence of active thymic tissue in the ectopic mediastinum. However, neither thymic nor ectopic fixation is associated with remission of the disease [29].

6. PRE-OPERATIVE PREPARATION

It is generally accepted that surgery should be offered to patients with myasthenia gravis, except for those with positive anti-MUSK antibodies, in whom it would be ineffective. Surgery improves the prognosis and the course of the disease, especially if it is performed early.Several studies have reported the efficacy of surgery in the treatment of myasthenia with complete thymic resection, despite the absence of prospective studies formally demonstrating the efficacy of thymectomy in myasthenia [30-32]. There is therefore a problem of indication for surgery in myasthenia without an associated thymic mass.Optimal management of patients with myasthenia gravis undergoing thymectomy is necessary. Good and careful pre-operative preparation should be carried out for all patients [33]. This pre-operative preparation includes :

o An assessment of autoimmune disorders

o Assessment of respiratory disorders

o Evaluation of cardiac function

o Optimising medical management of myasthenia gravis

6.1. Medical treatment

6.1.1. Cholinesterase inhibitors :

For the treatment of myasthenia, only Pyridostigmine bromide (Mestinon®) and Ambenonium chloride (Mytelase®) have marketing authorisation [34]. These treatments are started as soon as myasthenia is suspected. The onset of action is 30 minutes, with an overall duration of action of 4 hours. An overdose with the appearance of muscarinic syndrome may be observed at doses higher than 8 tablets (480mg/d) of Mestinon, which should always be investigated.

6.1.2. Immunotherapy :

6.1.2.1. Short-term immunotherapy :

It includes plasma exchange and intravenous immunoglobulin. It is indicated in cases of acute and severe relapses, including attacks of severe myasthenia. It may also be indicated prior to surgical resection in cases of myasthenia that are poorly balanced and/or symptomatic despite medical treatment.

➢ **Plasma exchanges**: The number of plasma exchanges and the time between exchanges varies according to the clinical response. It varies between 2 and 4 on average over 1 to 3 weeks.

➢ **Cures of immunoglobulins**: these are administered at a dose of 0.4g/Kg over 5 days, with a total dose of 2g/Kg [35].

6.1.2.2. Long-term immunotherapy :

It is indicated as soon as clinical signs are not improved by the usual anti-cholinesterase agents. First-line treatment is usually based on either corticosteroids (1mg/Kg/d Prednisone or Prednisolone) or Azathioprine (Imurel®) at a dose of 2-3mg/Kg/d, or a combination of both treatments [36] (Figure 7). In the event of ineffective or inadequately controlled myasthenia under corticosteroid therapy and/or Azathioprine, other immunosuppressive treatments may be proposed, such as Rituximab [37] (anti CD20 monoclonal antibody), Ciclosporin, and Cyclophosphamide (Endoxan®) [38].

6.1.3. Analgesics :

Level 1 analgesics are indicated to combat pain secondary to muscle weakness, mainly in the spinal column (leading to cervical pain which can be disabling).

6.1.4. Physiotherapy:

Re-training and muscle-building movements are contraindicated in cases of myasthenia. However, a gradual return to walking is recommended.for these patients in order to combat the de-training secondary to the disease.

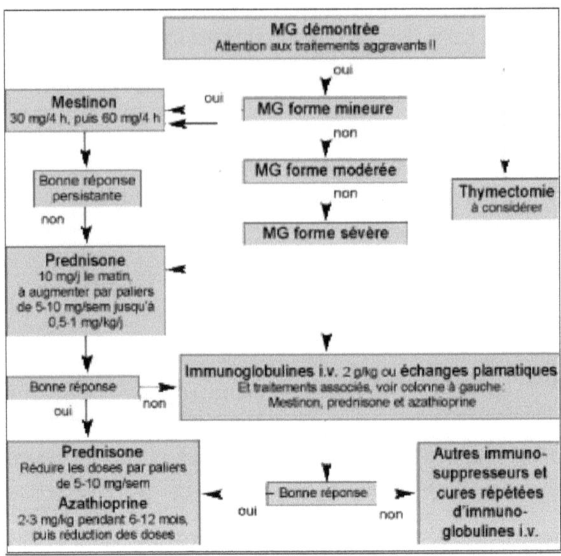

Figure 7: Summary of the overall management of Myasthenia Gravis

7. INDICATIONS FOR SURGERY

Surgical resection of the thymus (Thymectomy) is indicated for [5, 39] :

✓ All patients with myasthenia gravis except those with positive anti-MUSK antibodies (surgery ineffective in this case).

✓ All patients with a thymic tumour associated w i t h   myasthenia gravis

✓ Myasthenia resistant to the usual symptomatic treatments.

✓ All patients with myasthenia gravis under the age of 50.

✓ Patients with ocular myasthenia gravis, given the risk of progression to myasthenia gravis (which occurs in almost half of cases).

✓ Patients with ocular myasthenia associated with a thymic tumour, or who are resistant to the usual medical treatment.

The proposed surgical procedure should be a thymectomy (resection of the entire thymic gland) combined with resection of the cervicomediastinal and pericardial fat. The latter should be performed systematically in all patients with myasthenia gravis, given the marked improvement in clinical signs after re-operation of the patients and additional removal of cervicomediastinal fat, which may contain ectopic thymic tissue reported by Masaoka et al. since 1982 [40].

De Perrot et al. reported in their study that a complete surgical resection should include en-bloc resection of the thymus and all the fat situated between the lower pole of the thyroid glands above, the diaphragm below, the pleura laterally, the sternum anteriorly, and the pericardium posteriorly [41].

The various possible locations of ectopic thymic tissue throughout the mediastinal fat (Figure 8) have been described in :

o Extra-capsular mediastinal lobes

o From the lower pole of the thyroid

o In cervical fat

o Retrothyroid

o Innominate venous trunk

o Accessory cervical lobes

o Fat in the aortic-pulmonary window

o Mediastinal fat

o Cervico-cervico-mediastinal lobes

o Fat along the phrenic nerves

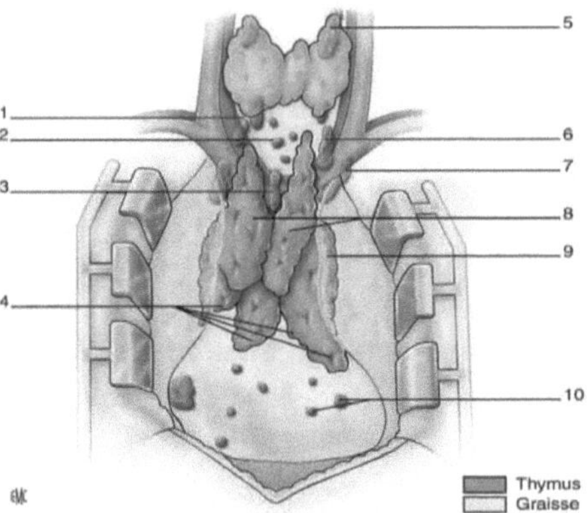

Figure 8: Schematic representation of the possible locations of ectopic thymic tissue in the mediastinum and mediastinal fat [30].

8. SURGICAL TREATMENT

8.1. Anaesthesia :

Good preparation with perioperative anaesthetic management of patients is essential. It should include :

- Proper assessment of autoimmune, respiratory and/or cardiac pathologies that may be associated with myasthenia [33].

- A continuation of treatmentmedical by anti-cholinesterase daily until the day before surgery.

- Plasma exchange sessions or courses of intravenous immunoglobulin, especially in cases of severe myasthenic crisis.

- During anaesthesia, particular attention is paid to avoiding the use of curares, which could aggravate the disease and lengthen the duration of the anaesthetic.

the length of hospitalisation. Other studies have also reported that muscle relaxant drugs can be used safely, provided that neuromuscular transmission is closely monitored intraoperatively [42]. The use of intermediate-acting non-depolarising muscle relaxants (such as atracirium and vecuronium) is possible, since their duration of action is rapid and completely reversible at the end of the operation.

- Particular attention must be paid to postoperative care, in order to achieve a :
❖ Essential pain relief

❖ Respiratory management, as well as postoperative mechanical ventilation, which may be necessary in severe cases of myasthenia gravis
❖ Appropriate titration and reversible elimination of muscle-relaxing anaesthetic drugs
❖ Management of anti-cholinesterase drugs

8.2. Surgical approaches :

Various surgical approaches have been described in the literature for performing a more or less enlarged thymectomy, depending on the clinical and radiological presentations of myasthenia gravis. We can distinguish :

8.2.1. Thymectomy by median sternotomy :

This is the most frequently used approach for resections that are mainly enlarged or for large tumours. The patient is positioned supine with a block under the shoulders, with the head slightly hyperextended and the arms at the side of the body or in a crook. A wide drape is used, extending from the neck to the umbilical region. The skin incision is median, running from the sternal fork to the xyphoid appendix. The sternum is opened vertically in the middle using a jigsaw or oscillating saw (Figure 9).

Dissection is performed from bottom to top, freeing the thymus from the pericardium and then from the vessels and venous plane, with ligation of the thymic veins. The pleura is pushed back on either side, and the phrenic nerves are located and avoided during dissection.

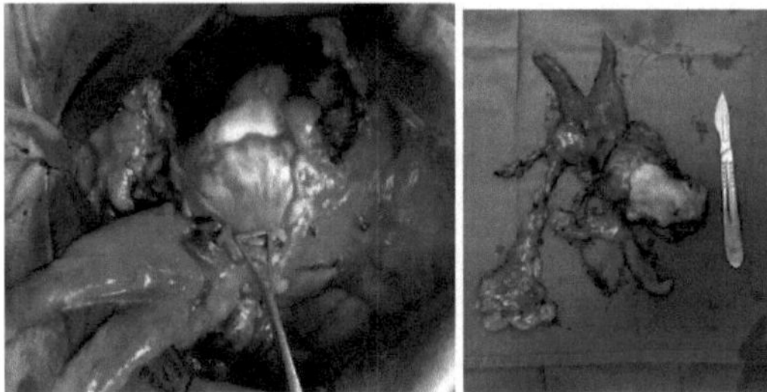

Figure 9: Thymectomy extended to the pleura by median sternotomy: Masaoka-Koga stage IIB thymoma (B2 60%, B3 10% and B1 30%).

For several teams, median sternotomy remains the surgical approach of choice for radical treatment of myasthenia gravis, to achieve total resection of the thymic gland combined with total removal of mediastinal fat and/or invaded adjacent structures (Figure 10).

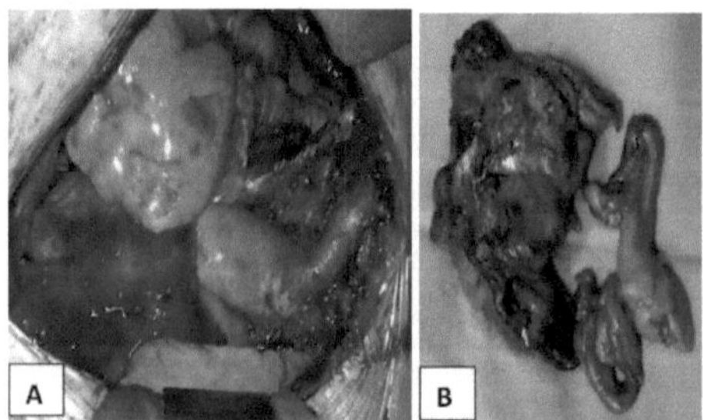

Figure 10 : Thymectomy extended to the right lung, phrenic nerve, innominate venous trunk and superior vena cava via median sternotomy.

Data on published series reporting surgical treatment of MG via median sternotomy are summarised in Table II below:

Table II: Median sternotomy thymectomies in the literature

Authors	Duration study	Nb patients	Age	Thymoma	Morbidity	Mortality	Improvement
Inderbitzi et al [43]. 1991	1986-1989	27		3 (11%)	0%	0%	77%
Hussain et al [44] 2010	2005-2009	22 (16F/6H)	35.2+/-14.5 years	4 (18.1%)			86.3%
Seyfari et al [45] 2018	2011-2016	47 (21F/26H)	33+/-4.6 years	40 (85.1%)	4.25% (mediastinitis + phrenic paralysis)	2.12%	85.1%
Kas et al [46] 2019	1985-2019	1002 (3.5F/1H)	32 (8-73 years old)	12.7%	respiratory distress (12.7%) mediastinitis (0.4%) bleeding (0.2%)	1.4%	

M: Men / F: Women / Nb: Number /

8.2.2. Thymectomy by cervicotomy :

The patient is positioned supine, with arms at his sides and venous access to each territory of the vena cava system. A block is placed under the shoulder blade with hyper-extension of the head. The drape should be wide, leaving the entire sternal region accessible for possible enlargement or conversion. The skin incision is made two fingerbreadths above the sternal fork in a fold of the neck. Removal will be gradual, gradually freeing the gland from top to bottom, looking for the thymic veins which drain into the inominate venous trunk, which should be clipped. This approach can be widened by opening the sternal manubrium (manubriotomy), giving better access to the thymic region and facilitating subsequent resection.Surgical resection of the thymus by the cervical route has been described and used by numerous teams. The first trans-cervical thymectomy for myasthenia gravis was performed by Crile in 1966 [47]. Total resection and extraction of the thymus by the cervical route is possible, but sometimes, in the presence of friable thymic tissue, enlargement by sternotomy or mini manubriotomy has been necessary to complete the operation.Crucitti et al. reported in a personal study carried out in 1977 on 75 patients operated on for myasthenia, that the group of patients operated on via the cervical approach only (36 patients) had a significantly shorter or even zero duration of postoperative respiratory assistance, compared with the group of patients operated on via the median sternotomy [48]. This cervical approach was excellent for the surgical treatment of myasthenia gravis, except in the case of thymic tumour masses, or in patients who had already been tracheostomised preoperatively. The cervicotomy technique was almost abandoned in favour of sternotomy, before Cooper described an improved technique of trans-cervical thymectomy through a 4-centimetre incision and after suspension of the sternal manubrium in 1988 [49]. No postoperative drainage was required, with an acceptable postoperative course and reduced length of stay compared with median sternotomy.

Nevertheless, cervicotomy has certain limitations [50] :
✓ There is a risk of incomplete resection of thymic tissue, with the possibility of leaving thymic remnants in place, which may lead to a lack of clinical improvement in the myasthenia postoperatively, and consequently to repeat surgery [40].

✓ Surgical technique difficult to learn, teach and adopt by as an effective and reproducible approach.

✓ Impossible of resection of large masses thymic masses sometimes associated with myasthenia by cervical approach only
✓ Cosmetic damage for large cervical incisions.

8.2.3. Trans-sternal and trans-cervical thymectomies:

The sternotomy may be extended upwards by an arched cervicotomy or opposite the sternocleidomastoid muscle. This approach is rarely used for thymic resection.

8.2.4. Video-assisted thymectomy:

The patient may be positioned in the left lateral decubitus, right lateral decubitus or dorsal decubitus position, depending on the approach chosen (right approach, left approach or bilateral videothoracoscopy). A block is usually placed under the shoulder blades with the arm raised at 90°. The surgeon sits on the patient's back with the monitor in front of him. He may use 3 or 4 trocars arranged in a triangle or diamond shape in the axillary region. The use of a 30° optic and CO2 insufflation could be beneficial for better exposure and dissection of the thymic gland. Once the mediastinal pleura has been opened, the entire mediastinal tissue is resected, starting from the pericardium and extending towards the retro-sternal region. While avoiding the phrenic nerves, dissection of the gland is carried out gradually until the innominate venous trunk is reached and the thymic veins are clipped. The dissection is then extended towards the neck to free the two horns (Figures 11, 12).

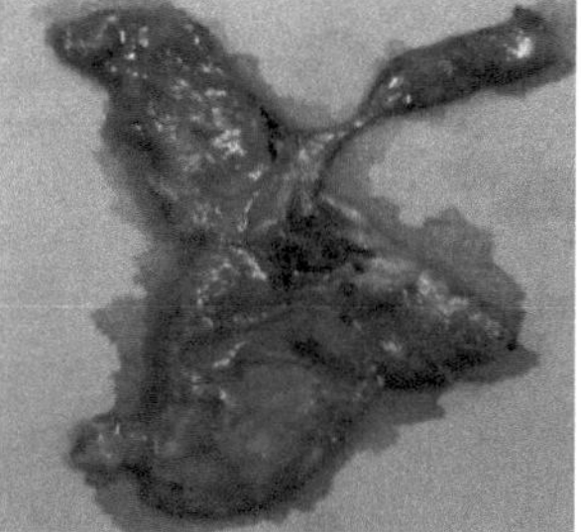

Figure 11: Thymectomy surgical specimen VATS: Thymic Hyperplasia

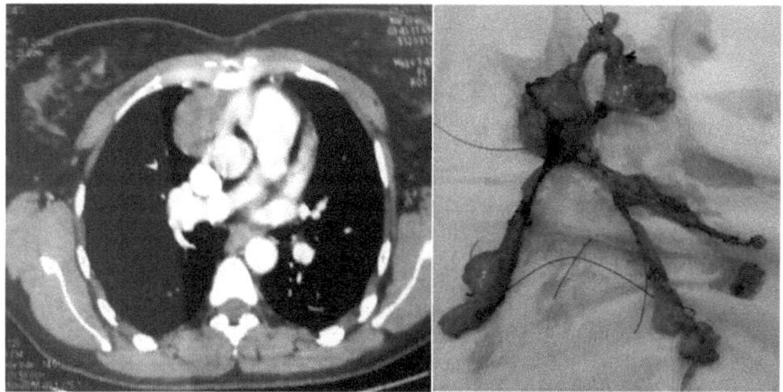

Figure 12: Thymectomy by right videothoracoscopy: B2 thymoma

With the advent of new minimally invasive techniques, particularly in thoracic surgery, thymectomy for myasthenia gravis has been described by several teams, with variations including the side (right or left approach), bilateral resections, and those via the subxyphoid approach. This approach reached its apogee following the introduction and use of selective intubation tubes, enabling single-lung ventilation with exclusion of the side being approached. The right side is most often used by several teams [50, 51]. The patient is placed in a 30° lateral decubitus position, with three trocars inserted, including one for the camera with a 30° optic. Insufflation of carbon dioxide makes this surgery much easier, as it facilitates exclusion of the ipsilateral lung, dissection of the tissue planes in the mediastinum, and visualisation of the cervical extension of the thymic gland. Drainage thoracic surgery may not be necessary at the end of the procedure, especially if there is no pulmonary wound. In his study, Tomulescu et al. found that the right and left approaches were similar in terms of operating time, length of hospital stay and remission rates [52]. In his opinion, the side approach is preferable because of the large amount of fat in the anterior mediastinum on the left side, which makes thymic dissection easier, the lower risk of injury to the right phrenic nerve because it is not in the operating field, and access to the aorto-pulmonary window if associated lymph node dissection is required. In comparing video-assisted thymectomy with other more invasive approaches, several studies have reported the advantage of this technique in terms of :

• Amount of blood lost during surgery

• Length of hospital stay

• Aesthetic result

• Reduced post-operative pain

• Easier return to work and social reintegration.

• Rapid mastery of the surgical technique, with an easy learning curve, and an easily reproducible operating technique unlike the trans-cervical technique.

However, video-assisted thymectomy does have its limitations, with the possibility of incomplete surgical resections, leaving thymic residues in place which may be associated with poorer post-operative results. To address the risk of incomplete resections with unremoved mediastinal thymic remnants, Novellino et al. reported in his study a technique that he named VATET (Videoassisted Thoracoscopic Extended Thymectomy) in order to be as radical as possible [53]. This technique combined a bilateral thoracoscopic approach with cervical exploration. The results of this approach in myasthenia gravis were reported by Mantegazza et al. with a 6-year follow-up of patients who had undergone thymectomy by sternotomy (47 patients) or by the VAVET technique (159 patients) [54]. Post-operative follow-up and complete remission rates were comparable in the two groups (50.6% versus 48.7% respectively in the sternotomy and VAVET resection groups). Similarly, the VAVET technique has been estimated to be better in terms of surgical resection of radical thymic tissue than cervicotomy alone [55]. Table III below summarises the results of video-assisted myasthenia gravis surgery compared or not with median sternotomy.

Table III: Surgery results for MG

Study	Wright et al (2002) [56]	Manlulu et al (2005) [57]	Bagheri et al (2018) [58]	Jurado et al (2012) [59]
Number	26	38	42	139 (13H/29F) Age 43 (34-51)
Comparative	No	No	Yes (21 VTS + 21 SM)	Yes (43 VATS + 96 SM)
Conversions	1/26		0/21	
Morbidity	1 phrenic paralysis	4	14.3% (VATS) 9.5% (SM) □ NR	9.1% (3 respiratory + 2 ACFA + 1 recurrent paralysis + 1 other)
Mortality	0%	0%	0%	0%
Stay (days)	4 (2-6)	3	0.73+/-4.67 (VATS) 0.97+/-5.95 (SM) □ 0.01	3 (3-5) : VATS 6 (5-8) : SM

M: Men / F: Women / SM: Median sternotomy / VATS: video-assisted thoracic surgery / VTS: videothoracoscopy / ACFA: atrial fibrillation arrhythmia / NS: Not reported

Minimally invasive surgery for myasthenia has been evaluated in the long term. In a series of 107 patients operated on using the minimally invasive technique, Tomulescu reported that patients were followed up more than one year after surgery [52]. His series was predominantly female (86%) and ranged in age from 8 to 60 years. The majority of patients were approached via the left approach (66%) with a morbidity of 9.34%, zero mortality, and an average hospital stay of 2.3 days (2-6 days). Mean follow-up was 3 years (12-74 months). During follow-up, no significant difference was demonstrated in terms of remission after surgery, length of hospital stay, morbidity and mortality, and anatomopathological results between patients operated on via the right or left approach. In terms of long-term follow-up and surgical results for myasthenia, Bachmann et al. reported in a long-term follow-up study of 106 patients followed for an average of 8 years (1-27 years) that the two approaches had the same result in terms of symptomatic improvement [60]. On the other hand, the minimally invasive techniques improved the signs associated with myasthenia better, reduced the total length of hospital stay, and caused less postoperative pain. This technique has even been presented as the reference approach for treating myasthenia gravis. This surgical attitude has also been adopted and confirmed by Comacchio [61] who indicated that for all early stage myasthenia gravis (with or without thymoma), minimally invasive techniques represent the surgical approach of choice with excellent oncological, neurological and surgical results. For advanced and locally invasive stages, a multi-disciplinary decision is required to choose the approach best suited to the patient and the associated thymic and loco-regional lesions.

8.2.5. Trans-cervical and sub-xyphoid thymectomies:

The patient is intubated with a selective tube. The patient is positioned supine, with a block under the shoulder blades and the head slightly hyperextended. The drape is wide, extending from the mandible to the umbilicus. During the cervical phase, the surgeon is positioned at the patient's head, and during the subxiphoid phase on the patient's right. Placement of a retractor under the sternal manubrium would allow upward sternal traction with better exposure of the anterior mediastinum. The subxiphoid stage is performed through an incision 4 to 6 cm below the xyphoid process, freeing it from the rectus abdominis muscles. A sternal retractor may also be used to improve exposure of the anterior mediastinum.

8.2.6. Subxyphoid thymectomy:

This approach is the same as that described above, combined with a trans-cervical approach, but without a neck approach.

8.2.7. Robot-assisted thymectomy (RATS) :

This approach uses the Da Vinci II robot, consisting of a control console with 3 or 4 articulated arms. Installation and draping are identical to those described for videothoracoscopy. Thymectomies are generally performed via 3 trocars: the first at the $3^{\text{ème}}$ intercostal space (ICS) on the anterior axillary line, the second at the $5^{\text{ème}}$ ICS on the anterior axillary line, and the third at the $5^{\text{ème}}$ ICS on the presternal line (Figure 13). This technique uses CO2 insufflation, which facilitates intraoperative dissection.Compared to videothoracoscopy, robotic thoracic surgery (especially after the introduction of the Da Vinci system) was introduced to remedy to the difficulties of videothoracoscopy and improve precision and manoeuvrability in the mediastinum during thymectomies (Figure 14).As with videothoracoscopy, the left-sided surgical approach has also been preferred for robotic surgery as reported by Augustin and colleagues on a series of 32 robot-assisted thymectomies in 2008 [62]. For this approach, the robotic camera is generally placed at the 6ème intercostal space on the middle axillary line, and the other two robotic arms are placed respectively at the 3ème and 6ème intercostal space.

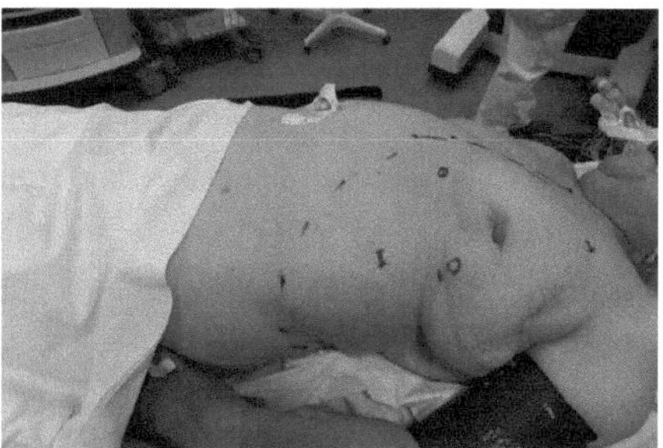

Figure 13: Patient positioning with trocar holes marked for the three robotic arms to be used (Charles Nicole University Hospital Rouen - France)

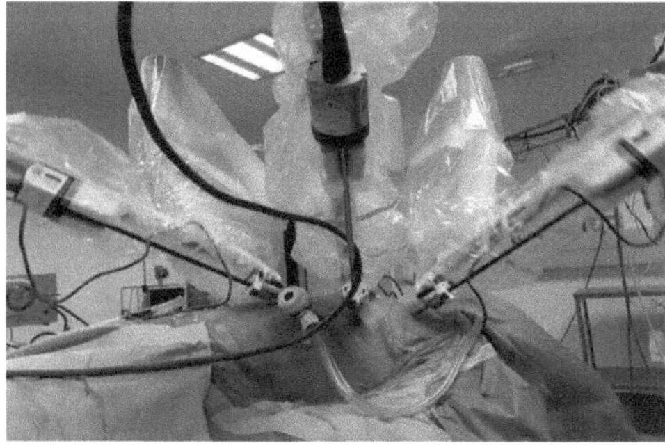

Figure 14: Robot-assisted left-axis thymectomy: intraoperative view positioning of trocars, robotic arms and camera with assistant trocar (Charles Nicole University Hospital Rouen - France)

The superiority of robotic surgery over other minimally invasive techniques has not yet been demonstrated in prospective randomised studies, but the robotic-assisted approach seems to be preferable, especially for enlarged thymectomies, because of the ease of dissection of the upper thymic horns (easier with carbon monoxide insufflation[63]), ligation of the thymic veins, and easier unilateral access to the entire anterior mediastinum [64].

In a French study based on the French national thoracic surgery database EPITHOR [65], a comparative study was carried out to evaluate the different techniques and surgical approaches for myasthenia gravis without thymoma. This study was conducted over a total period of 9 years and included a total of 278 patients divided into 3 groups (patients operated on by median sternotomy (47%), cervico-sternotomy (11%), and by videothoracoscopy or robotic approach in 42% of cases). No significant difference was demonstrated between the three groups studied, but a more frequent use of minimally invasive approaches was noted. Robot-assisted thymectomy for non-thymomatous myasthenias, or for myasthenias with an early stage thymoma (Masaoka- Koga stage I and II) currently represent the two indications of choice according to Li et al [66]. The left approach is better for anatomical reasons, especially for myasthenic patients, and even for repeat surgery in cases of refractory myasthenia despite initial thymectomy [67].

Kauppi et al even report that robot-assisted surgery for myasthenia gravis in young subjects who are well controlled on medical treatment is more likely to result in complete and stable remission in this type of patient [68].

Recently, a meta-analysis published in 2019 attempted to compare the results of thymectomy by the minimally invasive route, versus the conventional route by sternotomy. and the robotic approach [69]. According to this study, current data favour robotic surgery, which is better than open surgery and similar to minimally invasive surgery using videothoracoscopy. However, in the absence of prospective randomised studies, long-term follow-up is still required before any conclusions can be drawn regarding the oncological efficacy of this technique.

8.2.8. Single incision thymectomies (Uniportal VATS): After the advent of the technique of minimally invasive thoracic surgery through a single incision by Diego Gonzales Rivas in 2012, this technique was adopted and used by some teams, and thymectomy was described.

▪**Uni-portal trans-cervical thymectomy**: This technique was described by Lemaître et al. in 2019 using a basi-cervical incision one centimetre from the sternal forchette [70].

Once the two thymic horns have been dissected and placed on a retractor wire, a retractor is inserted and the thymus is dissected in an anterior plane from the sternal manubrium to the pericardium (Figures 15, 16, 17).

Careful dissection of the two lateral surfaces is then carried out before the entire gland is pushed forward, in order to clip the thymic veins once the inominate venous trunk has been identified. According to Lemaître, the morbidity associated with this technique is low (less than 2% in his series), with rare complications such as haemothorax, pneumothorax and surgical wound infection, but no reported damage to the recurrent nerve. The overall conversion rate remains below 1%.

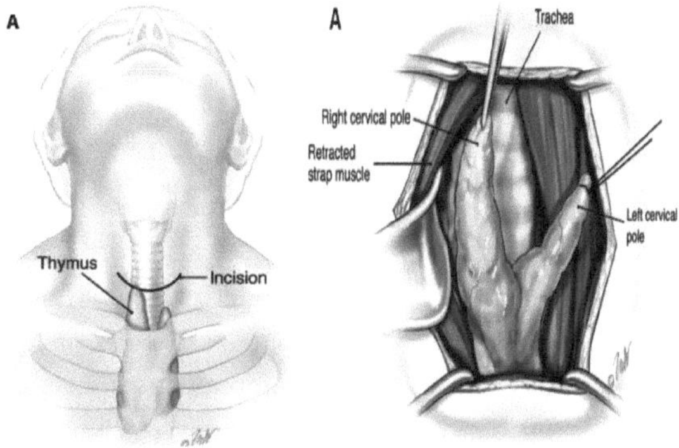

Figure 15: Cutaneous incision of the cervicotomy approach (A) and schematic representation of an intraoperative view of the thymus.

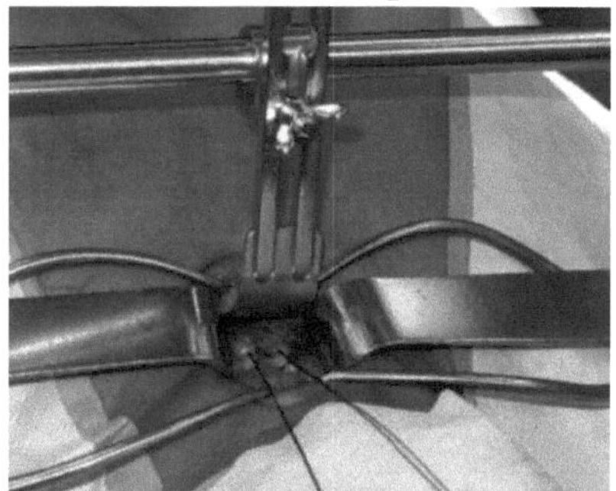

Figure 16: Intraoperative view of the exposed thymus gland

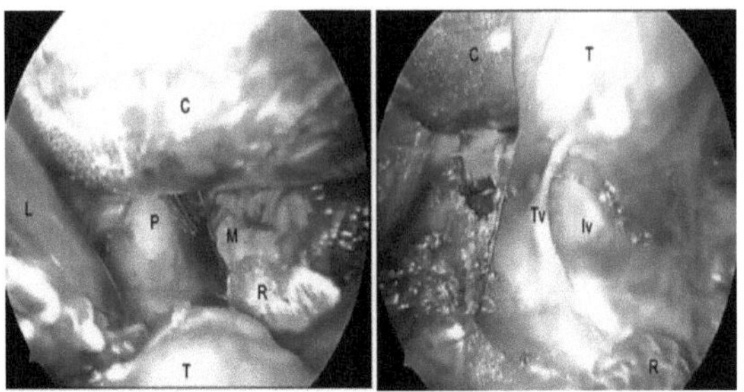

Figure 17: Endoscopic views of cervical thymectomy

- **Uni-portal thymectomy via the subxiphoid route:**

The subxyphoid approach to the thymus gland was described in 2001 by Uchiyama et al [71]. A sternal suspensor is inserted through a transverse subxyphoid incision, before a mediastinoscope is introduced through the subxyphoid incision (Figure 18). The authors reported a series of 23 patients with an overall conversion rate of 8.7% for carcinological reasons (need for further resection or poor exposure). Mortality was zero, with only one phrenic paralysis (an overall rate of 4.3%). Other technical modifications have been made to this approach. Indeed, in 2017, Zhong et al reported that a subxyphoid approach combined with a double VTS approach (one on each side) would avoid the phrenic nerve injuries described by Uchiyama, with fewer complications [72]. According to Aramini, the subxyphoid approach also has the advantage of reducing the possibility of intercostal nerve damage (often associated with VTS or RATS approaches), resulting in less post-operative pain, faster recovery with shorter hospital stay, and considerable aesthetic advantage [73]. In a comparative study of 107 patients [74], Xu et al. compared the post-operative course of patients who had undergone thymic resection via the subxiphoid route (37) versus lateral videothoracoscopy (70). The subxiphoid approach was correlated with shorter hospital stay, less postoperative pain and less intraoperative blood loss than the videothoracoscopic approach. In addition, for myasthenic patients, the subxiphoid approach had a significantly shorter operating time.

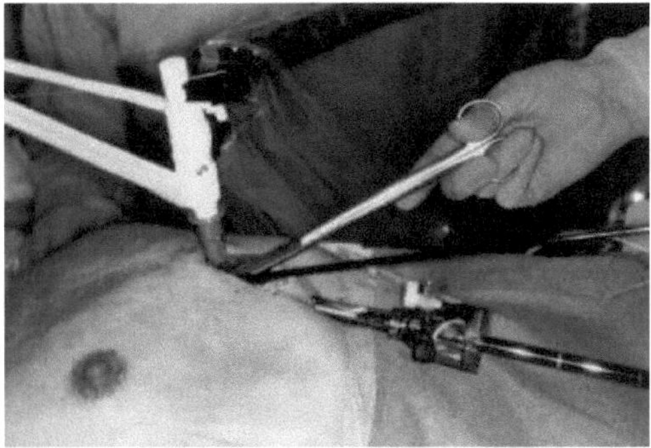

Figure 18: Intraoperative view of a subxiphoid approach for thymectomy

- **Robot-assisted thymectomy (RATS) via the subxiphoid approach:** Recently, this approach has also been used in robot-assisted surgery, either using two arms on either side (Figures 19, 20), or exclusively via a single-port approach, with all instruments passing through the same orifice.

RATS was performed on 13 patients, including 2 with myasthenia gravis, through a 4cm incision, with CO_2 insufflation, using 3 robotic arms and a 5mm curved cannula [75]. Mortality was zero and there were no major complications in this series.

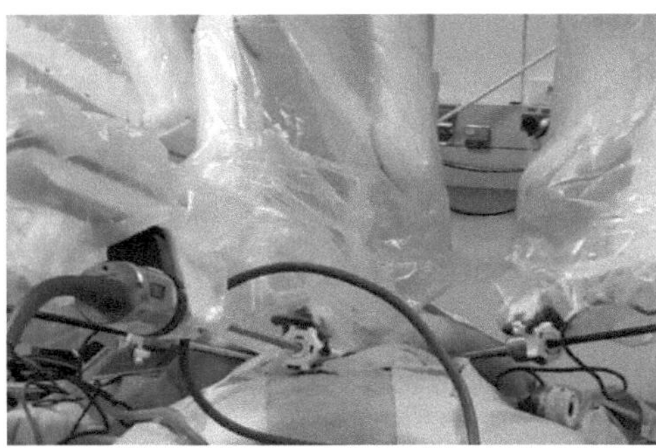

Figure 19: Robot-assisted subxiphoid approach with double thoracic approach (Charles Nicole University Hospital Rouen - France)

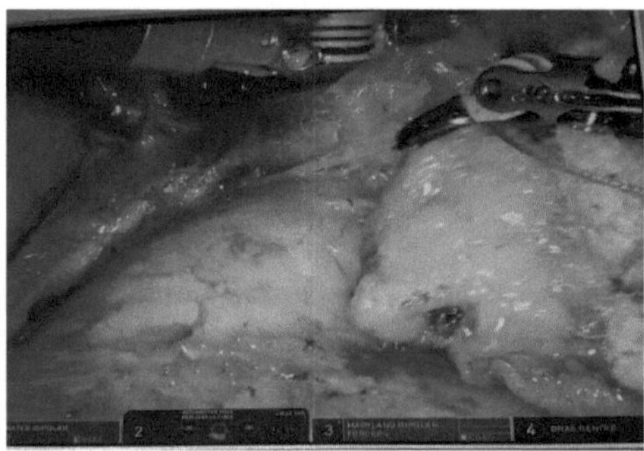

Figure 20: Endoscopic view of a subcutaneous robot-assisted thymectomy. xyphoid (vision in line with the elements of the mediastinum) (Charles Nicole University Hospital Rouen - France)

8.3. Operative gesture :

Principles of surgical resection in myasthenia gravis should include:
✓ Total resection of the thymus gland

✓ Resection of all pericardial and cervico-mediastinal fat that may contain thymic remnants.

✓ Particular care must be taken to preserve the integrity of the phrenic nerves as far as possible. Indeed, patients with myasthenia already have alveolar hypoventilation, which is likely to worsen if there is an associated phrenic lesion. This lesion is described in almost 7% of thymectomies.

✓ In the case of unilateral phrenic invasion: an overall benefit/risk assessment should be carried out for each case, especially in terms of possible respiratory complications depending on the patient's condition.

✓ In the case of bilateral invasion: one of the two phrenic nerves should be respected in order to avoid amputation of respiratory function as far as possible.

✓ Resection of the thymic tumour (if associated with myasthenia) because of its oncological prognosis, independently of the myasthenic disease.

9. POST-OPERATIVE CARE

9.1. Duration of intubation and hospitalisation in intensive care unit :

The optimal duration of intubation required postoperatively for thymectomy is unknown.In their study of 96 patients who had undergone thymectomy for myasthenia gravis, Chen et al. demonstrated that early extubation (before 6 hours post-op) was correlated with a statistically significant improvement in the post-op course, with fewer pneumopathies and a reduction in the total length of stay in the intensive care unit [76]. However, certain preoperative risk factors have been shown to prolong the duration of mechanical ventilation postoperatively, such as the MGFA clinical stage, myasthenia gravis not balanced under medical treatment, or at an advanced stage [77, 78].

9.2. Postoperative myasthenic seizures :

Myasthenic attacks after surgery are common, and a number of studies have looked into the subject.In fact, certain factors could play an important role in reducing the incidence of these attacks, such as the prescription of pre-operative plasmapheresis sessions in the case of a myasthenia-thymus tumour association [79], and the pre-operative administration of intravenous immunoglobulins for uncontrolled pre-operative myasthenic attacks [80].Wu et al. reported that prolonged administration of prostigmine, postoperative pulmonary infection, and the risk of developing a preoperative myasthenic crisis are risk factors for the development of a myasthenic crisis after thymectomy [81].Other risk factors have been identified by Li et al. such as the association with pre-operative bulbar signs and incomplete surgical resection of the thymoma.The development of a myasthenic crisis in the postoperative period would also be a risk factor. a poor prognostic factor for patients [82].

9.3. Prognostic factors in myasthenia gravis surgery :

The postoperative after-effects of myasthenia gravis surgery are all t h e more importantsimple as :

✓ Surgical resection is carried out early (within 6 months of the onset of the disease). the appearance of the first symptoms of the disease) [83].

✓ Sex is feminine

✓ Myasthenia is associated with dysthyroidism

✓ Preoperative myasthenia is serious [84].

✓ Age under 40

✓ The pathology is not thymomatous [85].

✓ Rehabilitation to postoperative exercise is early [86].

✓ Masaoka stage is more advanced or the occurrence of recurrence postoperatively [87].
✓ A minimally invasive approach is used [84].

10. POST-OPERATIVE THERAPEUTIC MANAGEMENT :

Surgical treatment is not the only cure for myasthenia gravis, but rather a link in a chain of comprehensive care. and multi-disciplinary. Complete resection of the thymus and all mediastinal fat is essential, without leaving any thymic residue, in order to improve post-operative management. Other therapeutic measures may be considered postoperatively:

10.1. Anti-cholinesterase treatment :

According to Kas et al. anti-cholinesterase treatment should be started as soon as possible, in order to avoid more respiratory complications [88]. In a population of 324 myasthenic patients operated on via median sternotomy, 71 (i.e. 22% of the total number of patients) presented respiratory complications, including 49 re-intubations or tracheostomies, following failure to introduce anti-cholinesterase treatment immediately after surgery. However, patients may show variable and random responses to anti-cholinesterase treatments, with a consequent reduced or even nil need for treatment. These may influence the ability to differentiate between myasthenic and cholinergic attacks, hence the argument for delayed or delayed resumption of treatment [42].

10.2. Postoperative analgesia :

It generally combines morphine (intravenous or epidural) with non-steroidal anti-inflammatory drugs. Epidural analgesia should be used with caution and with close monitoring of respiratory function, given the risk of respiratory depression, and should only be offered to patients operated via a sternotomy or thoracotomy [89].

10.3. Not recommended for myasthenic patients:

Certain treatments are likely to aggravate myasthenic syndromes,

It is therefore preferable to avoid them because of :
- Depression of the post-synaptic membrane and acetylcholine release:
Aminosides, Coistin, Clindamycin.
- Magnesium-rich solvent: tetracyclines for injection

- Potentiating effect of beta-blockers

- Risk of frequent complications from anti-epileptic drugs

10.4. Adjuvant treatments :

Particularly in cases of thymoma where pathological examination shows adhesions, capsular breakage and/or incomplete resection (not R0). Depending on the MASAOKA or GETT classification, adjuvant radiotherapy and/or chemotherapy may be proposed after discussion at a thoracic oncology multidisciplinary discussion meeting.

✓ Classification of the GETT Thymic Tumour Study Group :
In France, the GETT (Groupe d'étude des tumeurs thymiques) classification is often used. It defines four stages of the disease:

o Stage I Encapsulated tumour completely resected :

- IA without adhesions ;

- IB with adhesions

o Stage II Invasive tumour completely resected :

o Stage III Invasive tumour :

- IIIA Incomplete resection ;
- IIIB simple biopsy

o Stage IV :

- IVA supra-clavicular adenopathy, pleural graft ;

- IVB metastases

Stade	Critères diagnostique
I	Tumeur encapsulée totalement réséquée sans adhérences (IA) ou avec adhérences (IB)
II	Tumeur invasive complètement réséquée
III	Tumeur invasive avec résection incomplète (IIIA) ou simple biopsie (IIIB)
IV	Dissémination : ADP sus claviculaire ou greffe pleurale (IV A) ou Métastases (IV B).

✓ **Masaoka-Koga classification:** This is a clinical classification of thymomas which was first established by Akira Masaoka in 1981 and modified by Koga Kenji in 1994 (Figure 21). It allows clinical and microscopic staging based essentially on :
- **Stage I**: macroscopically completely encapsulated tumour, without capsular

invasion microscopy

- **Stage II**: macroscopic invasion of surrounding fatty tissue or mediastinal pleura, or microscopic capsular invasion.

- **Stage III**: macroscopic invasion of neighbouring organs (pericardium, lung, large vessels)

- **Stage IV** :

• Stage IVa: pleural or pericardial dissemination

• Stage IVb: lymph node metastases or distant metastases The Msaaoka-Koga classification represents the first classification of thymomas, with stages correlated with prognosis.

This classification is now the most widely used in the world since it was modified in 1994:

- **Stage I**: tumour completely encapsulated, macroscopically and microscopically

- **Stage II** :

• Stage IIa: microscopic transcapsular invasion

• Stage IIb: macroscopic invasion of the capsule or adipose tissue in contact, or macroscopic contact with the mediastinal pleura or pericardium without rupture of the latter

- **Stage III**: macroscopic invasion of neighbouring organs (pericardium, lung, large vessels)

- **Stage IV** :

• Stage IVa: pleural or pericardial dissemination

• Stage IVb: lymph node metastases or distant metastases

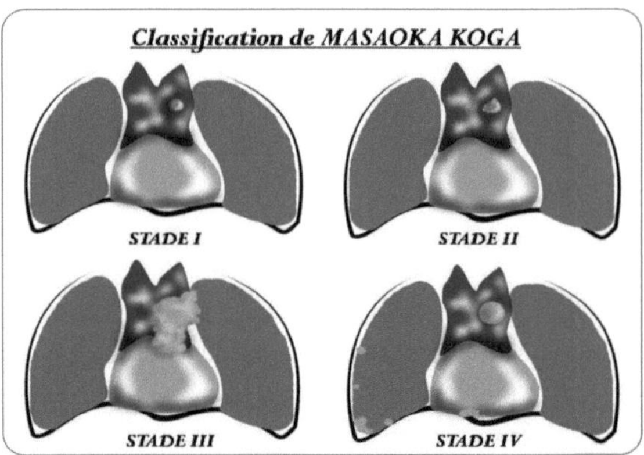

Figure 21: Schematic representation of the Masaoka-Koga classification

Management should be multidisciplinary, involving respirologists, neurologists, resuscitators, radiologists and surgeons. All cases of MG associated or not with a tumour of the thymic cavity should be discussed at the thoracic oncology multidisciplinary consultation meeting (RCP) or within a thymic tumour study team in order to reach a collegial decision (Figure 22).This RCP or thymic tumour study staff will also be responsible for discussing possible neo-adjuvant or adjuvant treatment after excision surgery, depending on the definitive anatomopathological stage (GETT or Masaoka- Koga classification) according to the diagram shown in Figure 23.

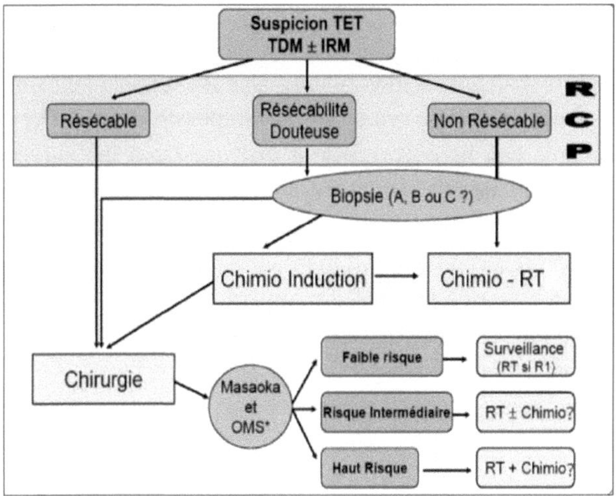

Figure 22: Diagram of management of tumours of the thymic cavity

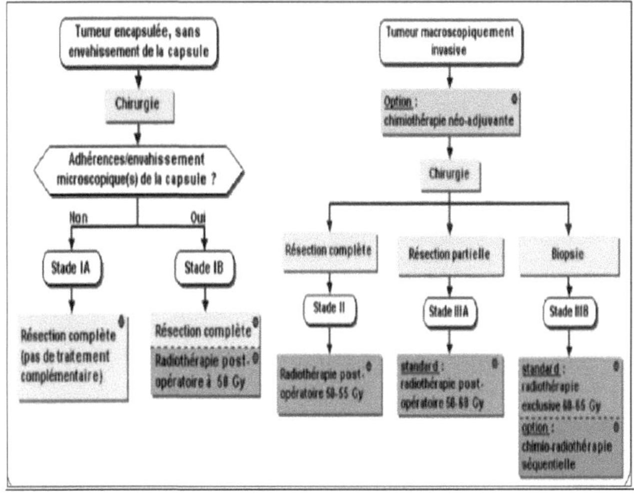

Figure 23: Diagram of management of thymic tumours according to anatomopathological stage and GETT classification

10.5. Tumour recurrence :

Although surgical resection markedly improves the clinical signs of myasthenia gravis, a late recurrence of the symptoms is still possible even after surgery [90]. In fact, myasthenia can be observed at a distance from the surgery, and even after revision of the thymic remnants left in place.Prolonged monitoring of myasthenic patients is therefore recommended in order to detect any clinical and/or radiological recurrences (thymic masses).Revision surgery should always be proposed as an effective option for treatment. The latter, with the presence of a recurrence-free survival interval are good prognostic factors in the event of thymoma recurrence [91].

11. EVOLUTION OF MG AFTER SURGICAL TREATMENT

The results of certain series reporting the evolution of MG after surgical resection are summarised in Table IV below:

Table IV: Evolution of MG after surgical treatment in the literature and in our series

	Wright et al (2002) [56]	Manlulu et al. (2005) [57]	Bagheri et al (2018) [58]
Number of patients	26	38	42
Progression of myasthenia gravis			
Improvement	81%	91.6%	90.5%
Stability	7.5%	5.2%	9.5%
Worsening	11.5%	3.2%	0%

The high peri-operative mortality rate could be explained by the fact that our series included patients with different histological types (notably lymphomas and thymic carcinomas) who were not included in the other studies.

12. MORBIDITY AND MORTALITY FACTORS

Despite the large number of studies reporting surgical results in myasthenia gravis, few have reported on morbidity and mortality factors. Table V below summarises the main studies that have reported risk factors for postoperative mortality and morbidity.

Table V: Studies reporting morbidity and mortality results after surgery for MG

Study	Ruffini et al [92]	Yu et al [93]	Wenxin et al [94]
Number	2030	178	194
Thymoma (%)	35 %	35%	100%
Average age	38	37	50
Morbidity factors	-Tumour size -Neuro-endocrine tumour -Incomplete resection - No thymoma	- Advanced age -Myasthenia score Pre-operative crisis -Thymoma	-Age -Masaoka Stadium -Clinical recurrence
Mortality factors	-Advanced age -Stage III, IV -Thymic carcinoma -Neuroendocrine tumour	-Bulbar syndrome -Duration of operation	-Bulbar syndrome (myasthenic crisis)

CONCLUSION

Myasthenia gravis (MG) is an autoimmune disease affecting the neuromuscular junction, responsible for the production of autoantibodies against acetylcholine receptors in striated skeletal muscle. Medical treatment is often combined with surgery to perform a simple or enlarged thymectomy. At present, it is generally accepted that surgical thymectomy should be proposed for all patients with MG except those with positive anti-MuSK antibodies.MG is a chronic disease, the treatment and follow-up of which is difficult because of its frequent and unpredictable fluctuations. Surgery for MG is currently indicated for any case of diagnosed myasthenia gravis, with or without an associated anterior mediastinal mass suggestive of a thymoma.Thymectomy therefore has a significant role to play in the management of MG, as a complement to the usual treatments administered. However, the risk of a myasthenic crisis occurring post-operatively, or of a worsening of symptoms necessitating an increase in and adaptation of medical treatments (anti-cholinesterase, corticosteroids, immunosuppressants, etc.) means that patients should always be well informed. New studies and series are increasingly favouring minimally invasive approaches to shorten the length of hospital stay and reduce postoperative pain, while respecting the rules of resection that is as complete as possible (involving the thymus gland and all mediastinal fat) and trying to preserve the integrity of the phrenic nerves.The earliest possible surgical management is therefore desirable, because the earlier patients are operated on, the better the post-thymectomy morbidity and mortality results.MG is associated with a higher morbidity and mortality rate when associated with a thymic tumour, with more clinical worsening postoperatively, which implies early surgical management in order to perform an enlarged thymectomy. Robotic surgery (RATS) is a technique of the future, better than videothoracoscopy in terms of complete resection and technical prowess, with results as good as minimally invasive approaches.

REFERENCES

1. Cataneo, A.J.M., G. Felisberto, Jr. and D.C. Cataneo, Thymectomy in nonthymomatous myasthenia gravis - systematic review and meta-analysis. Orphanet J Rare Dis, 2018. **13**(1): p. 99.

2. Robinson, C.L., The role of surgery of the thymus for myasthenia gravis. Ann R Coll Surg Engl, 1983. **65**(3): p. 145-51.

3. Blalock, A., et al, Myasthenia Gravis and Tumors of the Thymic Region: Report of a Case in Which the Tumor Was Removed. Ann Surg, 1939. **110**(4): p. 544-61.

4. Maggi, G., et al, Thymectomy in myasthenia gravis. Results of 662 cases operated upon in 15 years. Eur J Cardiothorac Surg, 1989. **3**(6): p. 504-9; discussion 510-1.

5. Osserman, K.E. and G. Genkins, Studies in myasthenia gravis: review of a twenty-year experience in over 1200 patients. Mt Sinai J Med, 1971. **38**(6): p. 497-537.

6. Masaoka, A., et al, Extended thymectomy for myasthenia gravis patients: a 20-year review. Ann Thorac Surg, 1996. **62**(3): p. 853-9.

7. Carr, A.S., et al, A systematic review of population based epidemiological studies in Myasthenia Gravis. BMC Neurol, 2010. **10**(46): p. 46.

8. Somnier, F.E., N. Keiding, and O.B. Paulson, Epidemiology of myasthenia gravis in Denmark. A longitudinal and comprehensive population survey. Arch Neurol, 1991. **48**(7): p. 733-9.

9. Berrih-Aknin, S. and R. Le Panse, [Myasthenia gravis and autoantibodies: Pathophysiology of the different subtypes]. Rev Med Interne, 2014. **35**(7): p. 413-20.

10. Aragones, J.M., et al, Myasthenia gravis: a higher than expected incidence in the elderly. Neurology, 2003. **60**(6): p. 1024-6.

11. Giraud, M., C. Vandiedonck, and H.J. Garchon, Genetic factors in autoimmune myasthenia gravis. Ann N Y Acad Sci, 2008. **1132**: p. 180-92.

12. Huang, D.R., et al, Tumour necrosis factor-alpha polymorphism and secretion in myasthenia gravis. J Neuroimmunol, 1999. **94**(1-2): p. 165-71.

13. Gregersen, P.K., et al, Risk for myasthenia gravis maps to a (151) Pro-->Ala change in TNIP1 and to human leukocyte antigen-B*08. Ann Neurol, 2012. **72**(6): p. 927-35.

14. Eymard, B., [Myasthenia, from the internist's point of view]. Rev Med Interne, 2014.**35**(7): p. 421-9.

15. Higuchi, O., et al, Autoantibodies to low-density lipoprotein receptor-related protein 4 in myasthenia gravis. Ann Neurol, 2011. **69**(2): p. 418-22.

16. Engstrom, J.W., Myasthenia gravis: diagnostic mimics. Semin Neurol, 2004. **24**(2): p. 141-7.
17. Newsom-Davis, J., Lambert-Eaton myasthenic syndrome. Rev Neurol (Paris), 2004.**160**(2): p. 177-80.

18. Klenczar, K., et al, [Myasthenia gravis, Graves-Basedow disease and other autoimmune diseases in patient with diabetes type 1 - APS-3 case report, therapeutic complications]. Pediatr Endocrinol Diabetes Metab, 2017. **23**(3): p. 159-164.

19. Engel, A.G., Current status of the congenital myasthenic syndromes. Neuromuscul Disord, 2012. **22**(2): p. 99-111.

20. Sanders, D.B., et al, A Double-Blinded, Randomized, Placebo-Controlled Trial to Evaluate Efficacy, Safety, and Tolerability of Single Doses of Tirasemtiv in Patients with Acetylcholine Receptor-Binding Antibody-Positive Myasthenia Gravis. Neurotherapeutics, 2015. **12**(2): p. 455-60.

21. Chan, K.H., et al, Frequency of seronegativity in adult-acquired generalized myasthenia gravis. Muscle Nerve, 2007. **36**(5): p. 651-8.

22. Oh, S.J., et al, Diagnostic sensitivity of the laboratory tests in myasthenia gravis.Muscle Nerve, 1992. **15**(6): p. 720-4.

23. Literature review of the usefulness of repetitive nerve stimulation and single fiber EMG in the electrodiagnostic evaluation of patients with suspected myasthenia gravis or Lambert-Eaton myasthenic syndrome. Muscle Nerve, 2001. **24**(9): p. 1239-47.

24. Nicholson, G.A., J.G. McLeod, and L.R. Griffiths, Comparison of diagnostic tests in myasthenia gravis. Clin Exp Neurol, 1983. **19**: p. 45-9.

25. Larner, A.J., The place of the ice pack test in the diagnosis of myasthenia gravis. Int J Clin Pract, 2004. **58**(9): p. 887-8.

26. Evoli, A., et al, Clinical correlates with anti-MuSK antibodies in generalized seronegative myasthenia gravis. Brain, 2003. **126**(Pt 10): p. 2304-11.

27. Priola, A.M. and S.M. Priola, Imaging of thymus in myasthenia gravis: from thymic hyperplasia to thymic tumor. Clin Radiol, 2014. **69**(5): p. e230-45.

28. Tuan, P.A., et al, The Value of CT and MRI for Determining Thymoma in Patients With Myasthenia Gravis. Cancer Control, 2019. **26**(1): p. 1073274819865281.

29. Mineo, T.C., V. Ambrogi, and O. Schillaci, May positron emission tomography reveal ectopic or active thymus in preoperative evaluation of non-thymomatous myasthenia gravis? J Cardiothorac Surg, 2014. **9**(146): p. 146.

30. Jaretzki, A., 3rd, Thymectomy for myasthenia gravis: analysis of controversies--patient management. Neurologist, 2003. **9**(2): p. 77-92.

31. Gronseth, G.S. and R.J. Barohn, Practice parameter: thymectomy for autoimmune myasthenia gravis (an evidence-based review): report of the Quality Standards Subcommittee of the American Academy of Neurology. Neurology, 2000. **55**(1): p. 7-15.

32. Sonett, J.R. and A. Jaretzki, 3rd, Thymectomy for nonthymomatous myasthenia gravis: a critical analysis. Ann N Y Acad Sci, 2008. **1132**: p. 315-28.

33. Krucylak, P.E. and K.S. Naunheim, Preoperative preparation and anaesthetic management of patients with myasthenia gravis. Semin Thorac Cardiovasc Surg, 1999. **11**(1): p. 47-53.

34. Mehndiratta, M.M., S. Pandey, and T. Kuntzer, Acetylcholinesterase inhibitor treatment for myasthenia gravis. Cochrane Database Syst Rev, 2014. **13**(10): p. CD006986.

35. Gajdos, P., S. Chevret, and K.V. Toyka, Intravenous immunoglobulin for myasthenia gravis. Cochrane Database Syst Rev, 2012. **12**(12): p. CD002277.

36. Palace, J., J. Newsom-Davis, and B. Lecky, A randomized double-blind trial

of prednisolone alone or with azathioprine in myasthenia gravis. Myasthenia Gravis Study Group. Neurology, 1998. **50**(6): p. 1778-83.

37. Nelson, R.P., Jr, et al, Rituximab for the treatment of thymoma-associated and de novo myasthenia gravis: 3 cases and review. J Clin Neuromuscul Dis, 2009. **10**(4): p. 170-7.

38. Sathasivam, S., Steroids and immunosuppressant drugs in myasthenia gravis. Nat Clin Pract Neurol, 2008. **4**(6): p. 317-27.

39. Ng, C.S., I.Y. Wan, and A.P. Yim, Video-assisted thoracic surgery thymectomy: the better approach. Ann Thorac Surg, 2010. **89**(6): p. S2135-41.

40. Masaoka, A., et al, Reoperation after transcervical thymectomy for myasthenia gravis.
Neurology, 1982. **32**(1): p. 83-5.

41. de Perrot, M. and K. McRae, Evidence for thymectomy in myasthenia gravis: Getting stronger? J Thorac Cardiovasc Surg, 2017. **154**(1): p. 314-316.

42. Baraka, A., Anesthesia and myasthenia gravis. Middle East J Anaesthesiol, 1993. **12**(1):p. 9-35.

43. Inderbitzi, R., K. Rosler, and B. Nachbur, [Trans-sternal thymectomy in myasthenia gravis]. Chirurg, 1991. **62**(6): p. 474-8.

44. Hussain, N., et al, Experience of thymectomy by median sternotomy in patients with myasthenia gravis. J Pak Med Assoc, 2010. **60**(5): p. 368-70.

45. Seyfari, B., et al, Clinical outcome of thymectomy in myasthenia gravis patients: A report from Iran. Iran J Neurol, 2018. **17**(1): p. 1-5.

46. Kas, J., et al, [Myasthenia gravis: perioperative complications of 1002 transsternal thymectomies - historical overwiev of 34 years long practice at one institution]. Magy Seb, 2019. **72**(3): p. 83-97.

47. Crile, G., Jr, Thymectomy through the neck. Surgery, 1966. **59**(2): p. 213-5.
48. Crucitti, F., F. Zucchetti, and G.B. Doglietto, [The cervical approach in surgery of the thymus for myasthenia. Comparison with the trans-sternal route. Considerations on 75 operated patients]. Minerva Chir, 1977. **32**(9): p. 543-7.

49. Cooper, J.D., et al, An improved technique to facilitate transcervical

thymectomy for myasthenia gravis. Ann Thorac Surg, 1988. **45**(3): p. 242-7.

50. Magee, M.J. and M.J. Mack, Surgical approaches to the thymus in patients with myasthenia gravis. Thorac Surg Clin, 2009. **19**(1): p. 83-9, vii.

51. Elsayed, H.H., et al, Video-assisted thoracoscopic thymectomy for non-thymomatous myasthenia gravis: a right-sided or left-sided approach? Interact Cardiovasc Thorac Surg, 2017. **25**(4): p. 651-653.

52. Tomulescu, V., et al, Thoracoscopic thymectomy mid-term results. Ann Thorac Surg, 2006. **82**(3): p. 1003-7.

53. Novellino, L., et al, "Extended" thymectomy, without sternotomy, performed by cervicotomy and thoracoscopic technique in the treatment of myasthenia gravis. Int Surg, 1994. **79**(4): p. 378-81.

54. Mantegazza, R., et al, Video-assisted thoracoscopic extended thymectomy (VATET) in myasthenia gravis. Two-year follow-up in 101 patients and comparison with the transsternal approach. Ann N Y Acad Sci, 1998. **841**: p. 749-52.

55. Shiono, H., N. Shigemura, and M. Okumura, Inclusion of the transcervical approach in video-assisted thoracoscopic extended thymectomy (VATET) for myasthenia gravis: a prospective trial. Surg Endosc, 2008. **22**(4): p. 1135-6.

56. Wright, G.M., S. Barnett, and C.P. Clarke, Video-assisted thoracoscopic thymectomy for myasthenia gravis. Intern Med J, 2002. **32**(8): p. 367-71.

57. Manlulu, A., et al, Video-assisted thoracic surgery thymectomy for nonthymomatous myasthenia gravis. Chest, 2005. **128**(5): p. 3454-60.

58. Bagheri, R., et al, Thymectomy for Nonthymomatous Myasthenia Gravis: Comparison of Video-Assisted Thoracoscopic and Transsternal Thymectomy. Innovations (Phila), 2018. **13**(2): p. 77-80.

59. Jurado, J., et al, Minimally invasive thymectomy and open thymectomy: outcome analysis of 263 patients. Ann Thorac Surg, 2012. **94**(3): p. 974-81; discussion 981-2.

60. Bachmann, K., et al, Long-term outcome and quality of life after open and thoracoscopic thymectomy for myasthenia gravis: analysis of 131 patients. Surg Endosc, 2008. **22**(11): p. 2470-7.

61. Comacchio, G.M., et al, Surgical Decision Making: Thymoma and Myasthenia Gravis. Thorac Surg Clin, 2019. **29**(2): p. 203-213.

62. Augustin, F., et al, Video-assisted thoracoscopic surgery versus robotic-assisted thoracoscopic surgery thymectomy. Ann Thorac Surg, 2008. **85**(2): p. S768-71.

63. Kaba, E., et al, Robotic thymectomy for myasthenia gravis. Ann Cardiothorac Surg, 2019. **8**(2): p. 288-291.

64. Savitt, M.A., et al, Application of robotic-assisted techniques to the surgical evaluation and treatment of the anterior mediastinum. Ann Thorac Surg, 2005. **79**(2): p. 450-5; discussion 455.

65. Orsini, B., et al, Comparative study for surgical management of thymectomy for non-thymomatous myasthenia gravis from the French national database EPITHOR. Eur J Cardiothorac Surg, 2016. **50**(3): p. 418-22.

66. Li, F., et al, Surgical Techniques for Myasthenia Gravis: Robotic-Assisted Thoracoscopic Surgery. Thorac Surg Clin, 2019. **29**(2): p. 177-186.

67. Li, F., et al, Robotic-Extended Rethymectomy for Refractory Myasthenia Gravis: A Case Series. Semin Thorac Cardiovasc Surg, 2019. **2**(19): p. 30332-6.

68. Kauppi, J., et al, Improvement in symptom remission rate following robotic thymectomy in patients with myasthenia gravis. Interact Cardiovasc Thorac Surg, 2020. **24**(5753902).

69. O'Sullivan, K.E., et al. A systematic review of robotic versus open and video assisted thoracoscopic surgery (VATS) approaches for thymectomy. Ann Cardiothorac Surg, 2019. **8**(2): p. 174-193.

70. Lemaitre, P.H. and S. Keshavjee, Uniportal Video-Assisted Transcervical Thymectomy. Thorac Surg Clin, 2019. **29**(2): p. 187-194.

71. Uchiyama, A., et al, Infrasternal mediastinoscopic thymectomy in myasthenia gravis: surgical results in 23 patients. Ann Thorac Surg, 2001. **72**(6): p. 1902-5.

72. Zhong, Y., et al, Modified Transsubxiphoid Thoracoscopic Extended Thymectomy in Patients with Myasthenia Gravis. Thorac Cardiovasc Surg, 2017. **65**(3): p. 250-254.

73. Aramini, B. and J. Fan, Technique for Myasthenia Gravis: Subxiphoid Approach.Thorac Surg Clin, 2019. **29**(2): p. 195-202.

74. Xu, H., et al, The Outcomes of Subxiphoid Thoracoscopic Versus Video-Assisted Thoracic Surgery for Thymic Diseases. J Laparoendosc Adv Surg Tech A, 2020. **31**(10).

75. Park, S.Y., et al, Subxiphoid approach for robotic single-site-assisted thymectomy. Eur J Cardiothorac Surg, 2020. **15**(5736520).

76. Chen, L., et al, Early extubation after thymectomy is good for the patients with myasthenia gravis. Neurol Sci, 2019. **40**(10): p. 2125-2132.

77. Lu, W., et al, Preoperative risk factors for prolonged postoperative ventilation following thymectomy in myasthenia gravis. Int J Clin Exp Med, 2015. **8**(8): p. 13990- 6.

78. Li, K.K., et al. Predictive factors of prolonged mechanical ventilation, overall survival, and quality of life in patients with post-thymectomy myasthenic crisis. World J Surg Oncol, 2017. **15**(1): p. 150.

79. Sarkar, B.K., P. Sengupta, and U.N. Sarkar, Surgical outcome in thymic tumors with myasthenia gravis after plasmapheresis--a comparative study. Interact Cardiovasc Thorac Surg, 2008. **7**(6): p. 1007-10.

80. Gamez, J., et al, Intravenous immunoglobulin to prevent myasthenic crisis after thymectomy and other procedures can be omitted in patients with well-controlled myasthenia gravis. Ther Adv Neurol Disord, 2019. **12**(1756286419864497): p. 1756286419864497.

81. Wu, Y., et al, Risk factors for developing postthymectomy myasthenic crisis in Thymoma Patients. J Cancer Res Ther, 2015. **11 Suppl 1**(1): p. C115-7.

82. Li, Y., et al, Clinical outcome and predictive factors of postoperative myasthenic crisis in 173 thymomatous myasthenia gravis patients. Int J Neurosci, 2018. **128**(2): p. 103-109.

83. Mineo, T.C. and V. Ambrogi, Outcomes after thymectomy in class I myasthenia gravis. J Thorac Cardiovasc Surg, 2013. **145**(5): p. 1319-24.

84. Kaufman, A.J., et al, Thymectomy for Myasthenia Gravis: Complete Stable Remission and Associated Prognostic Factors in Over 1000 Cases. Semin

Thorac Cardiovasc Surg, 2016. **28**(2): p. 561-568.

85. Kim, H., et al, Factors predicting remission in thymectomized patients with acetylcholine receptor antibody-positive myasthenia gravis. Muscle Nerve, 2018. **58**(6):p. 796-800.

86. Ambrogi, V. and T.C. Mineo, Benefits of Comprehensive Rehabilitation Therapy in Thymectomy for Myasthenia Gravis: A Propensity Score Matching Analysis. Am J Phys Med Rehabil, 2017. **96**(2): p. 77-83.

87. Tian, W., et al, Surgical effect and prognostic factors of myasthenia gravis with thymomas. Thorac Cancer, 2020. **19**(10): p. 1759-7714.

88. Kas, J., et al, Decade-long experience with surgical therapy of myasthenia gravis: early complications of 324 transsternal thymectomies. Ann Thorac Surg, 2001. **72**(5): p. 1691-7.

89. Kirsch, J.R., et al, Preoperative lumbar epidural morphine improves postoperative analgesia and ventilatory function after transsternal thymectomy in patients with myasthenia gravis. Crit Care Med, 1991. **19**(12): p. 1474-9.

90. Van Backer, J.T., A. Cedeno-Rodriguez, and J. Nabagiez, Third distant recurrence of benign thymoma in a patient with myasthenia gravis. BMJ Case Rep, 2019. **12**(4): p. 2018-228529.

91. Chiappetta, M., et al, Prognostic factors after treatment for iterative thymoma recurrences: A multicentric experience. Lung Cancer, 2019. **138**: p. 27-34.
92. Ruffini, E., et al, Tumours of the thymus: a cohort study of prognostic factors from the European Society of Thoracic Surgeons database. Eur J Cardiothorac Surg, 2014. **46**(3):p. 361-8.

93. Yu, L., et al, Thoracoscopic thymectomy for myasthenia gravis with and without thymoma: a single-center experience. Ann Thorac Surg, 2012. **93**(1): p. 240-4.

94. Tian, W., et al, Surgical effect and prognostic factors of myasthenia gravis with thymomas. Thorac Cancer, 2020. **11**(5): p. 1288-1296.

TABLE OF CONTENTS

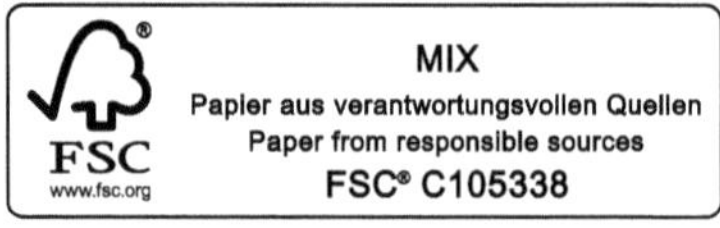

Printed by Books on Demand GmbH, Norderstedt / Germany